THE CANCER FIGHTING DIET

"Nourish, Move, thrive – Your Ultimate Guide to Deliciously Defending Against Cancer with Science, Fitness, and Heartfelt Support!"

ANNE FINLEY

Copyright © 2024

All Rights Are Reserved

The content in this book may not be reproduced, duplicated, or transferred without the express written permission of the author or publisher. Under no circumstances will the publisher or author be held liable or legally responsible for any losses, expenditures, or damages incurred directly or indirectly as a consequence of the information included in this book.

Legal Remarks

Copyright protection applies to this publication. It is only intended for personal use. No piece of this work may be modified, distributed, sold, quoted, or paraphrased without the author's or publisher's consent.

Disclaimer Statement

Please keep in mind that the contents of this booklet are meant for educational and recreational purposes. Every effort has been made to offer accurate, up-to-date, reliable, and thorough information. There are, however, no stated or implied assurances of any kind. Readers understand that the author is providing competent counsel. The content in this book originates from several sources. Please seek the opinion of a competent professional before using any of the tactics outlined in this book. By reading this book, the reader agrees that the author will not be held accountable for any direct or indirect damages resulting from the use of the information contained therein, including, but not limited to, errors, omissions, or inaccuracies.

TABLE OF CONTENTS

INTRODUCTION

In a world where the prevalence of cancer continues to rise, the pursuit of effective preventive measures and supportive treatments becomes paramount. "The Cancer-Fighting Diet" serves as a beacon of hope and practical guidance in navigating the intricate relationship between nutrition and cancer.

Cancer, a multifaceted and formidable adversary, demands a comprehensive approach to prevention and management. While medical advancements have made significant strides in the treatment landscape, the profound impact of dietary choices on cancer risk and progression cannot be overstated. This book is a testament to the transformative potential of embracing a purposeful and well-informed approach to nutrition.

Understanding the Role of Diet in Cancer Prevention

The journey toward a cancer-free life begins with knowledge. In the opening chapters, we delve into the fundamental principles of a cancer-fighting diet. We unravel the mysteries behind nutrient-rich foods, exploring the science of antioxidants and the potent role of phytochemicals in fortifying our bodies against the onslaught of cancerous cells. By establishing a solid foundation of understanding, readers will be empowered to make informed choices that resonate with the body's natural defence mechanisms.

The Basics of a Cancer-Fighting Diet

Building upon this foundation, we embark on a comprehensive exploration of the building blocks of a cancer-fighting diet. From the vibrant spectrum of fruits and vegetables to the essentiality of whole grains and lean proteins, we uncover the nutritional arsenal that can fortify the body's resilience. This section equips readers with the knowledge to create meals that not only satisfy the palate but also serve as powerful allies in the battle against cancer.

Superfoods for Cancer Prevention

Certain foods emerge as superheroes in the realm of cancer prevention. We spotlight the cruciferous vegetables with their potent anti-cancer properties, extol the virtues of berries as nature's formidable defenders, and explore the benefits of fatty fish rich in omega-3 fatty acids. Through this journey, readers will discover a curated list of superfoods that can be readily incorporated into their daily lives.

Creating Balanced Meals

Balancing nutrition is an art, and in this section, we guide readers through the intricate dance of crafting meals that are not only delicious but also nutritionally dense. From portion control to thoughtful meal planning, we empower individuals to take charge of their plates and, by extension, their health.

Hydration and Cancer

Amidst the array of dietary considerations, the role of hydration takes centre stage. We explore the significance of water in detoxification, highlight the potential benefits of herbal teas, and emphasize the importance of limiting sugary beverages. A well-hydrated body is better equipped to fend off the insidious threats posed by cancer.

Mindful Eating and Its Impact

Beyond the plate, we delve into the profound connection between mind and body. Mindful eating practices, stress reduction techniques, and the exploration of the mind-body connection become integral components of the cancer-fighting journey. This section invites readers to cultivate a holistic approach to well-being.

In the subsequent chapters, we navigate the nuanced terrain of nutritional support for cancer patients, offer a compendium of cancer-fighting recipes, and explore the symbiotic relationship between fitness and nutrition. This book is not just a guide; it is a compendium of empowerment, providing the tools and knowledge needed to embrace a cancer-fighting lifestyle.

CHAPTER ONE

THE BASICS OF A CANCER-FIGHTING DIET

Nutrient-Rich Foods

Let's take a thorough look at foods high in nutrients, keeping in mind their importance for human health and how they support different body functions.

Nutrient-Rich Foods: Nourishing the Human Body

The Essence of Nutrient-Rich Foods

Nutrient-rich foods form the bedrock of a healthy and vibrant life. These are foods that pack a powerful punch of essential vitamins, minerals, antioxidants, and other bioactive compounds that the human body requires for optimal functioning. In the pursuit of well-being, understanding and incorporating nutrient-rich foods into our diets is pivotal.

Key Components of Nutrient-Rich Foods:

1. *Vitamins and Minerals:* Nutrient-rich foods are abundant sources of vitamins and minerals essential for cellular function, immune response, and overall vitality. From vitamin A to zinc, each nutrient plays a unique role in maintaining health.

2. ***Antioxidants:*** These compounds combat oxidative stress and inflammation, key contributors to chronic diseases and aging. Fruits, vegetables, and certain nuts and seeds are rich sources of antioxidants, safeguarding cells from damage.

3. ***Fiber:*** Found in whole grains, legumes, fruits, and vegetables, fibre supports digestive health, regulates blood sugar levels, and contributes to a feeling of satiety.

4. ***Protein:*** Essential for the building and repair of tissues, proteins from both plant and animal sources are integral to a balanced diet. Nutrient-rich sources include lean meats, poultry, fish, eggs, dairy, legumes, and tofu.

5. ***Healthy Fats:*** Omega-3 and omega-6 fatty acids, found in fatty fish, nuts, seeds, and certain oils, support brain function, cardiovascular health, and inflammation regulation.

Humans as Nutrient Seekers

As creatures intricately woven into the fabric of nature, humans have evolved as nutrient seekers. Our bodies crave a diverse array of nutrients to function optimally, and the consumption of nutrient-rich foods aligns with our evolutionary history.

Bioavailability and Whole Foods:

The bioavailability of nutrients in whole foods surpasses that of isolated supplements. Whole foods provide a synergistic combination of nutrients, promoting better absorption and utilization by the body. Nature's packaging of nutrients in fruits, vegetables, whole grains, and lean proteins optimizes their delivery to our cells.

Customized Nutrient Needs:

Individual nutrient needs vary based on factors such as age, sex, activity level, and health status. Nutrient-rich foods cater to this diversity, offering a spectrum of essential compounds that can be tailored to meet individual requirements.

Incorporating Nutrient-Rich Foods into Everyday Life

Adopting a diet rich in nutrients need not be complex or restrictive. It involves making mindful choices and embracing a variety of whole, minimally processed foods. Consider the following strategies:

1. Diversify Your Plate:

- Include a colourful array of fruits and vegetables to ensure a spectrum of vitamins and minerals.

- Incorporate whole grains like quinoa, brown rice, and oats for fibre and essential nutrients.

2. Lean Proteins:

- Choose lean meats, poultry, fish, eggs, tofu, and legumes to meet protein needs.

3. Healthy Fats:

- Include sources of healthy fats such as avocados, nuts, seeds, and olive oil in moderation.

4. Mindful Cooking:

- Preserve the nutrient content of foods by opting for cooking methods like steaming, roasting, or sautéing instead of deep-frying.

5. Hydration Matters:

- Water is fundamental for nutrient transport and overall well-being. Ensure adequate hydration by incorporating water-rich foods and beverages.

Antioxidants and Their Impact on Cancer

Certainly! Now let's explore the function of antioxidants and how they affect cancer, emphasizing that humans produce antioxidants as a part of their defence systems.

Antioxidants and Their Crucial Role in Cancer Prevention

Antioxidants are a diverse group of compounds that play a pivotal role in protecting the body's cells from oxidative stress. Oxidative stress occurs when there is an imbalance between the production of reactive oxygen species (ROS) and the body's ability to neutralize them. ROS, including free radicals, are natural byproducts of various cellular processes, and while they have essential roles in signalling and immunity, an excess can lead to cellular damage.

Types of Antioxidants:

1. ***Endogenous Antioxidants:*** These are antioxidants that the body produces internally. They include enzymes like superoxide dismutase, catalase, and glutathione peroxidase, which work collectively to neutralize ROS.

2. ***Exogenous Antioxidants:*** Obtained from external sources, exogenous antioxidants come from the diet and include vitamins (such as vitamin C and E), minerals (like selenium and zinc), and various phytochemicals found in plants.

The Human Body as an Antioxidant Generator

Humans are equipped with a sophisticated antioxidant defense system that involves both endogenous and exogenous components. The body's ability to generate its antioxidants is a testament to its intricate design and the evolutionary imperative to combat oxidative stress.

Endogenous Antioxidant Enzymes:

1. *Superoxide Dismutase (SOD):* Converts superoxide radicals into less harmful molecules.

2. *Catalase:* Breaks down hydrogen peroxide into water and oxygen.

3. *Glutathione Peroxidase:* Utilizes glutathione to neutralize peroxides, protecting cells from damage.

Exogenous Antioxidants from the Diet:

1. *Vitamin C (Ascorbic Acid):* Found in fruits and vegetables, it scavenges free radicals and regenerates other antioxidants.

2. *Vitamin E (Tocopherols and Tocotrienols):* Present in nuts, seeds, and oils, it protects cell membranes from oxidative damage.

3. *Selenium:* Obtained from nuts, seeds, and seafood, it is a cofactor for various antioxidant enzymes.

4. **Flavonoids, Carotenoids, and Polyphenols:** Abundant in fruits, vegetables, and plant-based foods, these phytochemicals contribute to antioxidant defences.

Antioxidants and Cancer Prevention

1. Counteracting DNA Damage:

- Antioxidants play a crucial role in preventing DNA damage caused by oxidative stress. Unrepaired DNA damage can lead to mutations, a key factor in the development of cancer.

2. Inhibiting Cancer Cell Growth:

- Certain antioxidants have been found to inhibit the growth of cancer cells and reduce the risk of tumor formation.

3. Enhancing Immune Function:

- Antioxidants support immune function, aiding the body in recognizing and eliminating abnormal cells, including potentially cancerous ones.

4. Anti-Inflammatory Effects:

- Chronic inflammation is closely linked to cancer development. Antioxidants help mitigate inflammation, contributing to a cancer-protective environment.

5. Synergistic Effects:

- The synergy between endogenous and exogenous antioxidants creates a robust defense against oxidative stress, providing comprehensive protection against cancer initiation and progression.

Balancing Antioxidant Intake

While antioxidants offer profound health benefits, balance is key. Excessive intake of antioxidant supplements may disrupt the delicate balance of oxidative stress and compromise the body's natural defence mechanisms. Therefore, obtaining antioxidants through a varied and balanced diet is recommended.

Phytochemicals and Their Role in Cancer Prevention

Let's take a closer look at phytochemicals and their critical role in preventing cancer, highlighting the fact that people do not produce phytochemicals; instead, they get them from plant-based diets.

Phytochemicals: Nature's Cancer Warriors

Phytochemicals, also known as phytonutrients, are bioactive compounds found in plants. These natural compounds contribute to the vibrant colors, flavors, and disease-fighting properties of fruits, vegetables, whole grains, nuts, seeds, and other plant-based foods. While plants produce phytochemicals to protect themselves from environmental threats, humans can harness the power of these compounds to promote health and prevent diseases, including cancer.

Diversity of Phytochemicals:

1. *Flavonoids:* Present in fruits, vegetables, tea, and red wine, flavonoids exhibit antioxidant and anti-inflammatory properties.

2. *Carotenoids:* Found in orange, yellow, and green fruits and vegetables, carotenoids, including beta-carotene and lycopene, are potent antioxidants.

3. *Glucosinolates:* Abundant in cruciferous vegetables like broccoli and kale, glucosinolates have anti-cancer properties.

4. *Phenolic Acids:* Found in berries, nuts, and whole grains, phenolic acids contribute to antioxidant and anti-inflammatory effects.

5. *Saponins:* Present in legumes, whole grains, and some herbs, saponins have immune-boosting and anti-cancer properties.

The Human Diet as a Source of Phytochemicals

Unlike endogenous antioxidants that the human body produces internally, humans do not generate phytochemicals. Instead, we obtain these valuable compounds through the consumption of a diverse and colourful array of plant-based foods. The plant kingdom offers a treasure trove of phytochemical-rich options that contribute to our overall well-being.

Dietary Sources of Phytochemicals:

1. ***Fruits and Vegetables:*** Berries, citrus fruits, leafy greens, tomatoes, and cruciferous vegetables are rich in various phytochemicals.

2. ***Whole Grains:*** Brown rice, oats, quinoa, and whole wheat contain phenolic compounds with potential health benefits.

3. ***Nuts and Seeds:*** Almonds, walnuts, flaxseeds, and chia seeds provide a variety of phytochemicals.

4. ***Legumes:*** Beans, lentils, and peas are excellent sources of saponins and other phytochemicals.

5. ***Herbs and Spices:*** Turmeric, garlic, ginger, and cinnamon contain bioactive compounds with anti-inflammatory and anti-cancer properties.

Phytochemicals and Cancer Prevention

1. Antioxidant Properties:

- Phytochemicals act as antioxidants, neutralizing free radicals and reducing oxidative stress, a key factor in cancer development.

2. *Anti-Inflammatory Effects:*

- Many phytochemicals exhibit anti-inflammatory properties, helping to create an environment in the body that is less conducive to cancer growth.

3. Detoxification Support:

- Certain phytochemicals assist the body in detoxifying harmful substances, potentially reducing the risk of cancer.

4. *Regulation of Cell Growth:*

- Some phytochemicals influence cell signaling pathways, contributing to the regulation of cell growth and apoptosis (programmed cell death).

5. *Immune System Modulation:*

- Phytochemicals can modulate the immune system, enhancing its ability to recognize and eliminate cancer cells.

Embracing a Phytochemical-Rich Diet

1. *Colourful Plate:*

- Aim for a variety of colours on your plate, as different hues often indicate diverse phytochemical profiles.

2. Whole, Plant-Based Foods:

- Prioritize whole, minimally processed plant foods to maximize your intake of phytochemicals.

3. Culinary Herbs and Spices:

- Incorporate herbs and spices into your meals to not only enhance flavour but also boost your phytochemical intake.

4. Seasonal and Local Produce:

- Opt for seasonal and locally sourced fruits and vegetables to diversify your phytochemical intake.

CHAPTER TWO

BUILDING A STRONG FOUNDATION

The Power of Fruits and Vegetables

We should talk about the power of fruits and vegetables in detail, pointing out that people do not produce these things; instead, they obtain vital nutrients and health advantages by consuming them.

The Power of Fruits and Vegetables: Nature's Nutrient-Rich Treasure

Fruits and vegetables stand as vibrant emblems of health, providing a plethora of essential nutrients that contribute to overall well-being. These plant-based foods are rich in vitamins, minerals, fibre, antioxidants, and phytochemicals—elements that collectively form the foundation of a nutritious and disease-resistant diet.

Essential Nutrients Found in Fruits and Vegetables:

1. *Vitamins:* A spectrum of vitamins, including vitamin C, vitamin A, folate, and various B-vitamins, supports diverse bodily functions.

2. *Minerals:* Essential minerals such as potassium, magnesium, and calcium are abundant in fruits and

vegetables, contributing to heart health, bone strength, and overall vitality.

3. ***Dietary Fiber:*** Fruits and vegetables provide both soluble and insoluble fibre, supporting digestive health, regulating blood sugar levels, and promoting satiety.

4. ***Antioxidants:*** The antioxidant arsenal found in fruits and vegetables helps combat oxidative stress, reducing the risk of chronic diseases, including cancer.

5. ***Phytochemicals:*** These bioactive compounds, unique to plants, possess anti-inflammatory and cancer-preventive properties.

Humans and the Consumption of Fruits and Vegetables

Humans, being unable to generate fruits and vegetables, rely on their dietary choices to obtain the myriad benefits these foods offer. A diet abundant in fruits and vegetables is not just a culinary preference; it is a strategic investment in health.

Bioavailability of Nutrients:

1. ***Optimal Nutrient Absorption:*** The diverse array of nutrients found in fruits and vegetables is packaged in a way that enhances bioavailability, ensuring the body can absorb and utilize these compounds effectively.

2. ***Synergistic Effects:*** The combination of vitamins, minerals, fibre, antioxidants, and phytochemicals in whole fruits and vegetables creates a synergy that magnifies their health-promoting effects.

Health Benefits of Fruits and Vegetables

1. Cardiovascular Health:

- The potassium, fibre, and antioxidants in fruits and vegetables contribute to lower blood pressure, reduced cholesterol levels, and a healthier cardiovascular system.

2. Weight Management:

- The high fibre content in fruits and vegetables promotes a feeling of fullness, aiding in weight management by reducing overall calorie intake.

3. Digestive Health:

- Dietary fibre supports digestive regularity, prevents constipation, and may reduce the risk of colorectal cancer.

4. Immune Support:

- Vitamins such as C and A, along with various phytochemicals, bolster the immune system, enhancing the body's ability to defend against infections and illnesses.

5. Cancer Prevention:

- The unique compounds in fruits and vegetables, including antioxidants and phytochemicals, play a significant role in reducing the risk of certain cancers.

Practical Tips for Increasing Fruit and Vegetable Intake

1. Variety is Key:

- Consume a colourful variety of fruits and vegetables to ensure a broad spectrum of nutrients.

2. Seasonal and Local Choices:

- Opt for seasonal and locally sourced produce to maximize freshness and nutrient content.

3. Whole and Fresh:

- Choose whole, fresh fruits and vegetables over processed or canned options to preserve nutritional value.

4. Incorporate into Every Meal:

- Include fruits and vegetables in every meal and snack, making them a natural and habitual part of your diet.

5. *Creative Cooking Methods:*

- Experiment with different cooking methods—roasting, steaming, grilling—to retain flavors and nutrients.

Whole Grains for Optimal Health

Certainly! Let's take a close look at the significance of whole grains for good health, pointing out that although humans do not produce whole grains, they do gain a lot from eating them.

Whole Grains for Optimal Health: Harnessing the Nutritional Power

Whole grains are nutritional powerhouses, encompassing grains that retain their bran, germ, and endosperm. This contrast with refined grains, where the bran and germ are often removed, resulting in a loss of essential nutrients. Whole grains include varieties such as brown rice, quinoa, oats, barley, whole wheat, and bulgur.

Nutrient Composition of Whole Grains:

1. *Fiber:* Whole grains are rich in dietary fibre, including both soluble and insoluble fibre, promoting digestive health and regulating blood sugar levels.

2. *Vitamins and Minerals:* Whole grains provide a spectrum of vitamins (B vitamins, vitamin E) and

minerals (iron, magnesium, zinc) crucial for various physiological functions.

3. *Antioxidants:* The bran and germ of whole grains contain antioxidants that combat oxidative stress, contributing to overall well-being.

4. *Phytochemicals:* Whole grains contain unique phytochemicals with anti-inflammatory and antioxidant properties.

Humans and Whole Grains: A Synergetic Relationship

Humans do not generate whole grains; rather, we rely on the cultivation and processing of grains to incorporate them into our diets. The consumption of whole grains is integral to optimizing health, and our bodies have evolved to extract essential nutrients from these plant-based sources.

Digestive Benefits:

1. *Fiber and Digestive Regularity:* The fibre in whole grains promotes healthy digestion, preventing constipation and supporting a balanced gut microbiome.

2. *Blood Sugar Regulation:* The fibre content in whole grains helps regulate blood sugar levels, reducing the risk of insulin resistance and type 2 diabetes.

Cardiometabolic Health:

1. ***Cholesterol Management:*** Whole grains contribute to heart health by helping manage cholesterol levels, reducing the risk of cardiovascular diseases.

2. ***Weight Management:*** The satiating effect of whole grains supports weight management by promoting a feeling of fullness.

Disease Prevention:

1. ***Cancer Risk Reduction:*** Certain components in whole grains, including fibre and antioxidants, have been associated with a lower risk of certain cancers.

2. ***Chronic Disease Prevention:*** Regular consumption of whole grains is linked to a reduced risk of chronic diseases, including cardiovascular disease and certain metabolic disorders.

Incorporating Whole Grains into the Diet

1. Whole Grain Varieties:

- Include a variety of whole grains in your diet, such as quinoa, brown rice, whole wheat, barley, and oats.

2. Reading Labels:

- Check food labels to ensure products labeled as "whole grain" or "whole wheat" actually contain the entire grain.

3. Swap Refined Grains:

- Replace refined grains with whole grains in your meals, such as opting for whole grain bread, brown rice, or whole wheat pasta.

4. Breakfast Boost:

- Start your day with whole grain breakfast options like oatmeal, whole grain cereal, or whole wheat toast.

5. Snack Smart:

- Choose whole grain snacks, such as air-popped popcorn or whole grain crackers, for a satisfying and nutritious treat.

Lean Proteins and their Contribution to Cancer Prevention

Let us go over the importance of lean proteins and how they can help prevent cancer in detail, pointing out that humans cannot produce proteins on their own; instead, they must get them through diet.

Lean Proteins and Cancer Prevention: Building Blocks for Health

Proteins are fundamental macronutrients composed of amino acids, essential for building and repairing tissues, supporting immune function, and regulating various physiological processes. Lean proteins specifically refer to protein sources that are low in saturated fats and cholesterol, contributing to overall heart health and well-being.

Sources of Lean Proteins:

1. *Poultry:* Skinless chicken and turkey breast are examples of lean poultry.

2. *Fish:* Fatty fish such as salmon, trout, and tuna provide high-quality protein and omega-3 fatty acids.

3. *Lean Cuts of Meat:* Selecting lean cuts, such as sirloin or tenderloin, from beef or pork.

4. *Plant-Based Proteins:* Legumes, tofu, tempeh, edamame, and certain grains contribute to plant-based lean protein options.

Humans and Protein Intake: A Dietary Imperative

Humans do not generate proteins internally, underscoring the importance of obtaining these essential nutrients from dietary sources. Protein consumption is integral to supporting various bodily functions, and incorporating lean protein sources into the diet offers specific advantages for cancer prevention.

Protein Synthesis and Cellular Repair:

1. *Tissue Maintenance:* Proteins are crucial for the maintenance and repair of tissues, helping the body recover from injuries and stress.

2. *Immune Function*: Many immune system components, including antibodies, enzymes, and signalling molecules, are proteins. Adequate protein intake supports immune function, aiding the body in recognizing and eliminating abnormal cells.

Cancer Prevention Mechanisms:

1. *Cellular Regulation:* Proteins play a role in regulating cell growth, division, and apoptosis (programmed cell death), contributing to the prevention of abnormal cell proliferation.

2. *Antioxidant Enzymes:* Certain proteins, such as the antioxidant enzymes produced by the body, help counteract oxidative stress, a factor implicated in cancer development.

The Role of Lean Proteins in Cancer Prevention

1. Maintenance of Healthy Body Weight:

- Adequate protein intake, especially from lean sources, can contribute to weight management by promoting a feeling of fullness and supporting muscle mass.

2. Muscle Preservation:

- Lean proteins are essential for preserving muscle mass, particularly during periods of weight loss or illness. Maintaining muscle mass is crucial for overall health and functional capacity.

3. Omega-3 Fatty Acids from Fish:

- Fatty fish, a source of lean protein, also provides omega-3 fatty acids with anti-inflammatory properties that may contribute to cancer prevention.

4. Nutrient Density:

- Lean proteins are often nutrient-dense, providing not only high-quality protein but also essential vitamins and minerals that support overall health.

5. Reduction of Saturated Fats:

- Choosing lean protein sources helps reduce the intake of saturated fats, which is associated with a lower risk of certain cancers and cardiovascular diseases.

Practical Tips for Incorporating Lean Proteins

1. Diverse Protein Sources:

- Include a variety of lean protein sources in your diet to ensure a broad spectrum of essential amino acids.

2. Plant-Based Options:

- Incorporate plant-based proteins, such as legumes, tofu, and whole grains, to diversify your protein intake.

3. Mindful Cooking Methods:

- Choose healthy cooking methods, such as grilling, baking, or steaming, to retain the nutritional quality of lean proteins.

4. Balanced Meals:

- Create balanced meals that include lean proteins, whole grains, and a variety of colourful vegetables for a comprehensive nutrient profile.

5. Portion Control:

- Practice portion control to ensure that protein intake aligns with individual dietary needs and goals.

CHAPTER THREE

SUPERFOODS FOR CANCER PREVENTION

Cruciferous Vegetables and Their Anti-Cancer Properties

In order to fully utilize the potential health benefits of cruciferous vegetables—which are not produced by humans— take let's a thorough look at their anti-cancer characteristics.

Cruciferous Vegetables and Cancer Prevention: Nature's Protective Arsenal

Cruciferous vegetables belong to the Brassicaceae family and are characterized by their cross-shaped flowers. These nutrient-packed vegetables include:

1. *Broccoli*

2. *Cauliflower*

3. *Kale*

4. *Brussels Sprouts*

5. *Cabbage*

6. *Bok Choy*

7. *Turnips*

8. *Radishes*

Nutrient Profile:

1. *Glucosinolates:* Cruciferous vegetables contain glucosinolates, sulphur-containing compounds that give these vegetables their distinctive taste and aroma.

2. *Vitamins and Minerals:* Rich in vitamins C, K, and folate, as well as minerals like potassium and manganese.

3. *Fiber:* Contributing to digestive health and satiety.

4. *Antioxidants:* Contain various antioxidants, including carotenoids and flavonoids.

Humans and Cruciferous Vegetables: Dietary Allies in Cancer Prevention

Humans do not generate cruciferous vegetables but are reliant on their inclusion in the diet to benefit from their unique anti-cancer properties. The compounds found in cruciferous vegetables, particularly glucosinolates, undergo enzymatic breakdown when these vegetables are chopped, chewed, or digested. This breakdown results in the formation of bioactive compounds such as indoles, isothiocyanates, and sulforaphane, which contribute to the vegetables' anti-cancer effects.

Mechanisms of Anti-Cancer Properties:

1. **Detoxification and Elimination of Carcinogens:**

- Glucosinolates break down into isothiocyanates, which enhance the detoxification of carcinogens and support their elimination from the body.

2. **Cellular Protection and Apoptosis:**

- Sulforaphane, a potent compound found in broccoli, has been associated with inducing apoptosis (programmed cell death) in cancer cells and protecting normal cells from damage.

3. **Anti-Inflammatory Effects:**

- Cruciferous vegetables contain anti-inflammatory compounds that may reduce inflammation, a key factor in cancer development.

4. **Inhibition of Tumour Growth:**

- Indoles and isothiocyanates may inhibit the growth of tumours by regulating cell cycle progression and promoting the destruction of abnormal cells.

Cruciferous Vegetables and Specific Cancers

1. Breast Cancer:

- Studies suggest that cruciferous vegetable consumption may be associated with a reduced risk of breast cancer, possibly due to their impact on oestrogen metabolism.

2. Colorectal Cancer:

- Regular intake of cruciferous vegetables has been linked to a lower risk of colorectal cancer, with potential mechanisms including anti-inflammatory and anti-carcinogenic effects.

3. Prostate Cancer:

- Some studies indicate that cruciferous vegetables may have protective effects against prostate cancer, possibly through mechanisms involving hormonal regulation.

Practical Tips for Incorporating Cruciferous Vegetables

1. Varied Cooking Methods:

- Enjoy cruciferous vegetables raw, steamed, roasted, or sautéed to diversify your culinary experience and nutrient intake.

2. Pairing with Other Vegetables:

- Combine cruciferous vegetables with a variety of other vegetables to create balanced and flavourful dishes.

3. Include in Salads and Stir-Fries:

- Toss broccoli, cauliflower, or kale into salads or stir-fries for a nutrient-rich boost.

4. Experiment with Different Types:

- Explore less common cruciferous vegetables like bok choy, turnips, or radishes for variety in taste and nutritional content.

5. Regular Incorporation:

- Aim for regular inclusion of cruciferous vegetables in your weekly meal plans to ensure a consistent intake of their health-promoting compounds.

Berries: Nature's Cancer Fighters

Now let's take a closer look at how berries help prevent cancer, pointing out that in order to fully benefit from these special health features, humans must eat berries, as they are not produced by them.

Berries: Nature's Cancer Fighters

Berries, vibrant and bursting with flavour, belong to a diverse group of fruits that include strawberries, blueberries, raspberries, blackberries, and cranberries. These small but mighty fruits are packed with a plethora of bioactive compounds that contribute to their health-promoting properties.

Nutrient Profile:

1. ***Antioxidants:*** Berries are rich in antioxidants, including anthocyanins, flavonoids, quercetin, and resveratrol, which combat oxidative stress.

2. ***Vitamins and Minerals:*** Berries provide essential vitamins, particularly vitamin C, and minerals such as manganese.

3. ***Dietary Fiber:*** The fiber content in berries, including both soluble and insoluble fiber, supports digestive health and helps regulate blood sugar levels.

4. ***Phytochemicals:*** Bioactive compounds in berries, like polyphenols, contribute to their anti-inflammatory and anti-cancer properties.

Humans and the Inclusion of Berries: A Dietary Imperative

Humans do not generate berries, but our dietary choices determine our access to the health benefits these fruits offer. Including berries in our diets becomes a strategic and delicious way to tap into their unique cancer-fighting potential.

Mechanisms of Cancer Prevention:

1. ***Antioxidant Defence:***

   - Berries' rich antioxidant content helps neutralize free radicals, reducing oxidative stress and its potential role in cancer development.

2. ***Anti-Inflammatory Effects:***

   - The anti-inflammatory properties of berries may help create an environment less conducive to cancer initiation and progression.

3. ***Apoptosis Induction:***

   - Some compounds in berries have been associated with inducing apoptosis (programmed cell death) in cancer cells, preventing their uncontrolled growth.

4. *Inhibition of Angiogenesis:*

- Certain berries have demonstrated the ability to inhibit angiogenesis, the formation of new blood vessels that support tumour growth.

5. *Metabolic Regulation:*

- Berries may play a role in regulating metabolic processes, potentially impacting factors associated with cancer risk.

Berries and Specific Cancers

1. Breast Cancer:

- Studies suggest that the antioxidants and phytochemicals in berries may contribute to a reduced risk of breast cancer.

2. Colorectal Cancer:

- The dietary fiber and anti-inflammatory compounds in berries may have protective effects against colorectal cancer.

3. Prostate Cancer:

- Some research indicates that the polyphenols in berries may be associated with a lower risk of prostate cancer.

Practical Tips for Incorporating Berries

1. Daily Inclusion:

- Aim to include a variety of berries in your daily diet to maximize their health benefits.

2. Fresh or Frozen Options:

- Enjoy fresh berries when in season and consider frozen options, which retain their nutritional value and can be convenient year-round.

3. Smoothies and Parfaits:

- Incorporate berries into smoothies, yogurt parfaits, or breakfast bowls for a delicious and nutrient-packed start to your day.

4. Snacking and Desserts:

- Snack on a handful of berries or use them in desserts as a healthier alternative to sugary treats.

5. Berry Medleys:

- Create colourful and nutritious berry medleys by combining different types of berries for a synergistic nutrient boost.

Fatty Fish and Omega-3 Fatty Acids

Let's take a thorough look at the advantages of fatty fish and omega-3 fatty acids, highlighting the fact that although these are not produced by humans, they are essential nutrients that must be received through diet in order to maintain good health.

Fatty Fish and Omega-3 Fatty Acids: Nourishing the Body and Mind

Fatty fish, such as salmon, mackerel, trout, herring, and sardines, are nutritional powerhouses rich in omega-3 fatty acids. These essential fatty acids, particularly eicosapentaenoic acid (EPA) and docosahexaenoic acid (DHA), play vital roles in various physiological processes.

Nutrient Profile of Fatty Fish:

1. *Omega-3 Fatty Acids:* Especially EPA and DHA, which are polyunsaturated fats crucial for brain health, cardiovascular function, and overall well-being.

2. *Protein:* High-quality protein that provides essential amino acids necessary for tissue repair and maintenance.

3. *Vitamins and Minerals:* Rich in vitamins D and B12, as well as minerals like selenium.

4. *Astaxanthin:* A powerful antioxidant that gives some fatty fish, like salmon, their distinctive color and provides additional health benefits.

Humans and the Need for Omega-3 Fatty Acids

Humans do not generate omega-3 fatty acids internally, highlighting the importance of incorporating them into the diet. The benefits of omega-3 fatty acids extend beyond mere nutrition, impacting various aspects of health, from cardiovascular function to cognitive well-being.

Cognitive Health:

1. *Brain Development and Function:* DHA is a key component of brain cell membranes and plays a crucial role in cognitive development, especially in infants and young children.

2. *Mood Regulation:* Omega-3 fatty acids may contribute to mood regulation and have been associated with a reduced risk of depression.

Cardiovascular Health:

1. *Heart Protection:* EPA and DHA contribute to heart health by reducing triglyceride levels, lowering blood pressure, and preventing irregular heartbeats.

2. ***Anti-Inflammatory Effects:*** Omega-3 fatty acids have anti-inflammatory properties, reducing inflammation in blood vessels and minimizing the risk of cardiovascular diseases.

Joint Health:

1. ***Reduced Inflammation:*** Omega-3s may alleviate joint pain and stiffness by reducing inflammation, benefiting individuals with conditions like arthritis.

Cancer Prevention:

1. ***Potential Anti-Cancer Effects:*** Some studies suggest that omega-3 fatty acids may have anti-cancer properties, although more research is needed in this area.

Incorporating Fatty Fish into the Diet

1. Regular Consumption:

- Aim to include fatty fish in your diet at least two times a week to meet omega-3 fatty acid requirements.

2. Variety of Choices:

- Explore different types of fatty fish to diversify your nutrient intake. Salmon, mackerel, trout, and sardines are excellent choices.

3. Grilled or Baked Preparations:

- Opt for healthier cooking methods like grilling or baking to retain the nutritional benefits of fatty fish.

4. Omega-3 Supplements:

- Consider omega-3 supplements, particularly if it's challenging to incorporate sufficient fatty fish into your regular meals.

5. Mindful Sourcing:

- Choose wild-caught fish whenever possible, as they may have higher omega-3 content compared to farm-raised varieties.

CHAPTER FOUR

CREATING BALANCED MEALS

Crafting Nutrient-Dense Meals

This is a detailed discussion on the importance of cooking nutrient-dense meals, emphasizing that while humans cannot synthesize nutrients on their own, we do require a well-balanced diet to sustain optimal health.

Crafting Nutrient-Dense Meals: A Blueprint for Human Vitality

Nutrient density refers to the concentration of essential nutrients—such as vitamins, minerals, proteins, and fibre—in a given portion of food in relation to its calorie content. Crafting meals with high nutrient density is pivotal for ensuring that the human body receives the necessary building blocks for optimal function and well-being.

Components of Nutrient-Dense Meals:

1. ***Colourful Vegetables and Fruits:*** Packed with vitamins, minerals, and antioxidants.

2. ***Whole Grains:*** Rich in fibre, B-vitamins, and essential minerals.

3. ***Lean Proteins:*** Providing high-quality amino acids for tissue repair and maintenance.

4. ***Healthy Fats:*** Incorporating sources like avocados, nuts, and olive oil for essential fatty acids.

5. ***Dairy or Dairy Alternatives:*** Supplying calcium, vitamin D, and other vital nutrients.

Humans and the Need for Nutrient-Dense Meals

Humans do not generate essential nutrients internally; therefore, the composition of our diets plays a fundamental role in meeting our nutritional requirements. Crafting meals that are nutrient-dense ensures that our bodies receive a balanced array of vitamins, minerals, and other essential components necessary for optimal health.

Energy and Nutrient Synergy:

1. ***Metabolic Function:*** Nutrient-dense meals provide the energy necessary for metabolic processes, supporting cellular function and overall vitality.

2. ***Cognitive Health:*** Essential nutrients contribute to brain health, impacting cognitive function, memory, and mood regulation.

3. ***Immune Support:*** Adequate vitamins and minerals are crucial for a robust immune system, helping the body defend against infections and illnesses.

4. ***Bone Health:*** Calcium, vitamin D, and other minerals from nutrient-dense foods contribute to bone strength and density.

Crafting Nutrient-Dense Meals: Practical Tips

1. Colourful Plate:

- Aim for a diverse and colourful array of vegetables and fruits to ensure a broad spectrum of nutrients.

2. Whole, Unprocessed Foods:

- Prioritize whole, unprocessed foods to maximize nutrient content and minimize empty calories.

3. Balanced Macronutrients:

- Include a balance of carbohydrates, proteins, and healthy fats in each meal to support various bodily functions.

4. Mindful Portion Control:

- Be mindful of portion sizes to avoid overconsumption and maintain a healthy balance of nutrients.

5. *Hydration:*

- Water is an essential component of nutrient transport and various physiological processes. Ensure adequate hydration.

6. *Culinary Creativity:*

- Experiment with herbs, spices, and healthy cooking methods to enhance flavor without compromising nutritional value.

Portion Control and Its Significance

I want to take this opportunity to go over the importance of portion management in detail. I want to emphasize that although humans do not create portion sizes, controlling and regulating the amount of food consumed is essential to leading a healthy and balanced life.

Portion Control: Mastering the Art of Balanced Eating

Portion control involves managing the size of food servings to ensure a balanced intake of calories and nutrients. This practice is essential for maintaining a healthy weight, preventing overeating, and optimizing nutritional intake. While humans do not generate portion sizes, developing an awareness and understanding of appropriate portions is a key aspect of promoting overall well-being.

Components of Portion Control:

1. ***Balanced Meals:*** Dividing the plate to include appropriate portions of proteins, carbohydrates, vegetables, and fats.

2. ***Mindful Eating:*** Paying attention to hunger and fullness cues to avoid unnecessary overconsumption.

3. ***Caloric Awareness:*** Understanding the caloric content of foods and adjusting portions based on individual dietary needs and goals.

4. ***Healthy Snacking:*** Portioning out snacks to prevent mindless eating and excessive calorie intake.

Humans and the Need for Portion Control

While humans do not generate portion sizes inherently, the modern food environment often provides larger portions than necessary. Controlling portion sizes becomes crucial in managing energy intake, supporting weight management, and ensuring a well-rounded intake of essential nutrients.

Energy Balance:

1. ***Weight Management:*** Portion control helps individuals maintain a healthy weight by preventing excess calorie consumption.

2. ***Metabolic Health:*** Proper portion sizes contribute to balanced energy intake, supporting metabolic processes and overall health.

Nutritional Adequacy:

1. ***Balanced Nutrient Intake:*** Portion control allows for a more balanced distribution of macronutrients and micronutrients across meals.

2. ***Preventing Nutrient Imbalances:*** Avoiding excessive intake of certain nutrients, such as sugars or saturated fats, supports overall health and reduces the risk of chronic diseases.

Behavioural Aspects:

1. **Cognitive Awareness:** Practicing portion control cultivates mindfulness, encouraging individuals to be more aware of what and how much they eat.

2. **Preventing Overeating:** Smaller portions can help prevent overeating, allowing individuals to enjoy a variety of foods without consuming excessive calories.

Portion Control Strategies: Practical Tips

1. Use Visual Cues:

- Familiarize yourself with visual cues like the size of a palm or a deck of cards to estimate appropriate portion sizes for proteins.

2. Choose Smaller Plates:

- Opt for smaller plates to create the illusion of a fuller plate, promoting satisfaction with smaller portions.

3. Be Mindful of Snacking:

- Portion out snacks in advance to avoid continuous grazing and mindless eating.

4. Listen to Hunger Cues:

- Pay attention to your body's hunger and fullness signals to guide portion sizes.

5. Share Larger Portions:

- When dining out, consider sharing larger portions with a friend to avoid overeating.

6. Read Nutrition Labels:

- Utilize nutrition labels to understand serving sizes and make informed decisions about food choices.

Meal Planning for Cancer Prevention

Let's examine meal planning in detail as a means of preventing cancer, pointing out that although people do not naturally create certain meal plans, the decisions we make about how to arrange our meals are vital in maintaining good health and lowering the risk of cancer.

Meal Planning for Cancer Prevention: A Holistic Approach to Well-Being

Meal planning involves thoughtful consideration of the foods and nutrients included in one's daily or weekly meals. While humans do not generate specific meal plans instinctively, the act of planning meals strategically contributes to overall health, including cancer prevention.

Components of Cancer-Preventive Meal Planning:

1. ***Inclusion of Anti-Inflammatory Foods:*** Incorporating foods with anti-inflammatory properties.

2. ***Balanced Macronutrients:*** Ensuring a balanced distribution of carbohydrates, proteins, and healthy fats.

3. ***Abundance of Fruits and Vegetables:*** Prioritizing a variety of colourful fruits and vegetables rich in antioxidants and phytochemicals.

4. ***Limiting Processed Foods:*** Minimizing the intake of processed and refined foods associated with an increased risk of cancer.

Humans and the Influence of Meal Choices on Cancer Prevention

While humans do not inherently generate specific meal plans, the dietary choices we make directly impact our susceptibility to various health conditions, including cancer. Meal planning for cancer prevention involves selecting foods that provide essential nutrients, antioxidants, and other bioactive compounds associated with reducing the risk of cancer.

Nutritional Factors:

1. ***Antioxidant Defence:*** Including foods rich in antioxidants helps neutralize free radicals, reducing oxidative stress implicated in cancer development.

2. ***Fiber Intake:*** A diet high in fibre, derived from whole grains, fruits, and vegetables, supports digestive health and may reduce the risk of certain cancers.

3. ***Healthy Fats:*** Choosing sources of healthy fats, such as those found in fatty fish, avocados, and nuts, contributes to overall well-being.

4. ***Phytochemicals:*** Selecting a variety of plant-based foods ensures a diverse intake of phytochemicals, which may have protective effects against cancer.

Lifestyle Factors:

1. ***Maintaining Healthy Weight:*** Meal planning that supports weight management reduces the risk of obesity-related cancers.

2. ***Regular Physical Activity:*** Combining meal planning with regular exercise contributes to a holistic approach to cancer prevention.

Dietary Patterns:

1. ***Mediterranean Diet:*** Embracing a Mediterranean-style diet, rich in fruits, vegetables, whole grains, and olive oil, has been associated with a lower risk of certain cancers.

2. ***Plant-Based Diets:*** Plant-based diets, emphasizing fruits, vegetables, legumes, and whole grains, have shown promise in reducing the risk of various cancers.

Practical Tips for Cancer-Preventive Meal Planning

1. Colourful Plate:

- Prioritize a variety of colourful fruits and vegetables to ensure a diverse range of nutrients and antioxidants.

2. Whole Grains:

- Choose whole grains such as brown rice, quinoa, and whole wheat, providing fibre and essential nutrients.

3. Lean Proteins:

- Incorporate lean proteins from sources like poultry, fish, legumes, and tofu to support tissue repair and immune function.

4. Healthy Fats:

- Include sources of healthy fats, such as avocados, olive oil, and nuts, while minimizing saturated and trans fats.

5. Limit Processed Foods:

- Reduce the intake of processed and red meats, sugary beverages, and highly processed snacks.

6. Hydration:

- Stay adequately hydrated with water and limit the consumption of sugary drinks.

7. Mindful Eating:

- Practice mindful eating by paying attention to hunger and fullness cues, avoiding overeating.

CHAPTER FIVE

RECIPES FOR A CANCER-FIGHTING LIFESTYLE

Breakfast Recipes

These ten breakfast dishes for cancer-fighting diets include ingredients, preparation and serving times, nutritional data, instructions, and two ways to serve.

1. Berry Blast Smoothie Bowl

Ingredients:

- 1 cup mixed berries (blueberries, strawberries, raspberries)
- 1 banana
- 1/2 cup Greek yogurt
- 1 tablespoon chia seeds
- 1 tablespoon honey
- 1/2 cup granola

Prep Time: 5 minutes

Serving Time: 10 minutes

Nutritional Info (per serving):

- Calories: 352

- Protein: 16g

- Fiber: 7g

- Antioxidants: High

Instructions:

1. Blend mixed berries, banana, Greek yogurt, and chia seeds until smooth.

2. Pour the smoothie into a bowl.

3. Top with honey and granola.

4. Serve chilled.

Serving Methods:

- Garnish with additional fresh berries.

- Add a sprinkle of flaxseeds for extra fibre.

2. Avocado and Smoked Salmon Toast

Ingredients:

- 1 slice whole-grain bread

- 1/2 ripe avocado, mashed

- 2 oz smoked salmon

- 1 teaspoon lemon juice

- Fresh dill for garnish

- Salt and pepper to taste

Prep Time: 10 minutes

Serving Time: 5 minutes

Nutritional Info (per serving):

- Calories: 240

- Protein: 14g

- Omega-3 Fatty Acids: High

Instructions:

1. Toast the whole-grain bread slice.

2. Spread mashed avocado on the toast.

3. Arrange smoked salmon on top.

4. Drizzle with lemon juice and season with salt and pepper.

5. Garnish with fresh dill.

Serving Methods:

- Serve with a side of mixed greens.

- Add a poached egg on top for extra protein.

3. Quinoa Breakfast Bowl

Ingredients:

- 1/2 cup cooked quinoa

- 1/4 cup almond milk

- 1 tablespoon chia seeds

- 1/2 cup mixed berries

- 1 tablespoon almond butter

- 1 teaspoon honey

Prep Time: 15 minutes

Serving Time: 10 minutes

Nutritional Info (per serving):

- Calories: 310

- Protein: 13g

- Fiber: 8g

- Antioxidants: High

Instructions:

1. Mix cooked quinoa with almond milk and chia seeds.

2. Let it sit for 10 minutes to thicken.

3. Top with mixed berries, almond butter, and honey.

Serving Methods:

- Sprinkle with sliced almonds for added crunch.

- Mix in a scoop of protein powder for an extra protein boost.

4. Turmeric and Ginger Oatmeal

Ingredients:

- 1/2 cup old-fashioned oats

- 1 cup almond milk

- 1/2 teaspoon turmeric powder

- 1/2 teaspoon grated ginger

- 1 tablespoon honey

- Fresh fruit for topping

Prep Time: 10 minutes

Serving Time: 5 minutes

Nutritional Info (per serving):

- Calories: 279

- Protein: 9g

- Anti-Inflammatory Compounds: High

Instructions:

1. Cook oats in almond milk until creamy.

2. Stir in turmeric powder and grated ginger.

3. Sweeten with honey and top with fresh fruit.

Serving Methods:

- Sprinkle with ground flaxseeds for added fibre.

- Serve with a dollop of Greek yogurt for extra protein.

5. Spinach and Feta Omelette

Ingredients:

- 2 eggs

- 1 cup fresh spinach, chopped

- 2 tablespoons feta cheese, crumbled

- 1/4 cup cherry tomatoes, diced

- 1 teaspoon olive oil

- Salt and pepper to taste

Prep Time: 10 minutes

Serving Time: 7 minutes

Nutritional Info (per serving):

- Calories: 221

- Protein: 17g

- Vitamin A and K: High

Instructions:

1. Whisk eggs and season with salt and pepper.

2. Heat olive oil in a pan and sauté spinach until wilted.

3. Pour eggs into the pan, add tomatoes and feta.

4. Cook until the omelette is set, then fold and serve.

Serving Methods:

- Garnish with fresh herbs like parsley.

- Serve with a side of whole-grain toast.

6. Chia Seed Pudding with Mango

Ingredients:

- 2 tablespoons chia seeds

- 1/2 cup almond milk

- 1/2 teaspoon vanilla extract

- 1/2 cup diced mango

- 1 tablespoon shredded coconut

Prep Time: 5 minutes (+overnight chilling)

Serving Time: 5 minutes

Nutritional Info (per serving):

- Calories: 181

- Fiber: 7g

- Omega-3 Fatty Acids: Moderate

Instructions:

1. Mix chia seeds, almond milk, and vanilla extract in a jar.

2. Refrigerate overnight or for at least 4 hours.

3. Top with diced mango and shredded coconut before serving.

Serving Methods:

- Add a dollop of Greek yogurt for creaminess.

- Drizzle with honey for extra sweetness.

7. Sweet Potato and Kale Breakfast Hash

Ingredients:

- 1 medium sweet potato, diced

- 1 cup kale, chopped

- 1/2 red bell pepper, diced

- 2 eggs

- 1 tablespoon olive oil

- Paprika and garlic powder to taste

Prep Time: 15 minutes

Serving Time: 10 minutes

Nutritional Info (per serving):

- Calories: 319

- Protein: 11g

- Vitamin C: High

Instructions:

1. Heat olive oil in a skillet and sauté sweet potatoes until tender.

2. Add kale, bell pepper, paprika, and garlic powder.

3. Create two wells in the mixture and crack eggs into them.

4. Cover and cook until eggs are done to your liking.

Serving Methods:

- Top with avocado slices for creaminess.

- Serve with a side of whole-grain toast.

8. Almond and Blueberry Overnight Oats

Ingredients:

- 1/2 cup rolled oats

- 1/2 cup almond milk

- 1 tablespoon almond butter

- 1/4 cup blueberries

- 1 tablespoon honey

- Sliced almonds for topping

Prep Time: 5 minutes (+overnight chilling)

Serving Time: 5 minutes

Nutritional Info (per serving):

- Calories: 280

- Protein: 8g

- Antioxidants: High

Instructions:

1. Mix rolled oats, almond milk, almond butter, and blueberries in a jar.

2. Refrigerate overnight.

3. Drizzle with honey and top with sliced almonds before serving.

Serving Methods:

- Stir in a scoop of Greek yogurt for added protein.

- Sprinkle with ground flaxseeds for extra fiber.

9. Cucumber and Avocado Breakfast Wrap

Ingredients:

- 1 whole-grain wrap

- 1/2 avocado, sliced

- 1/2 cucumber, julienned

- 2 tablespoons hummus

- 1 tablespoon sunflower seeds

- Fresh mint leaves for garnish

Prep Time: 10 minutes

Serving Time: 5 minutes

Nutritional Info (per serving):

- Calories: 300

- Fiber: 11g

- Vitamin E: High

Instructions:

1. Spread hummus on the wrap.

2. Layer with avocado, cucumber, and sunflower seeds.

3. Garnish with fresh mint leaves.

4. Roll up the wrap and slice before serving.

Serving Methods:

- Serve with a side of mixed berries.

- Add a poached egg for extra protein.

10. Broccoli and Mushroom Frittata

Ingredients:

- 4 eggs

- 1 cup broccoli florets, blanched

- 1/2 cup mushrooms, sliced

- 1/4 cup feta cheese, crumbled

- 1 tablespoon olive oil

- Fresh herbs (such as thyme or parsley)

- Salt and pepper to taste

Prep Time: 15 minutes

Serving Time: 15 minutes

Nutritional Info (per serving):

- Calories: 283

- Protein: 15g

- Vitamin D: Moderate

Instructions:

1. Whisk eggs and season with salt and pepper.

2. Heat olive oil in an oven-safe pan and sauté mushrooms.

3. Add blanched broccoli and pour in the whisked eggs.

4. Sprinkle feta cheese and fresh herbs on top.

5. Bake in the oven until the frittata is set.

Serving Methods:

- Serve with a side of mixed greens.

- Top with a dollop of Greek yogurt for creaminess.

Lunch Recipes

Below are ten lunchtime cancer-fighting diet recipes, together with their components, preparation and serving times, nutritional data, guidelines, and two different ways to serve them.

1. Salmon and Quinoa Salad

Ingredients:

- 1 cup cooked quinoa
- 4 oz grilled salmon, flaked
- 1 cup mixed greens
- 1/2 cucumber, sliced
- 1/4 cup cherry tomatoes, halved
- 1 tablespoon olive oil
- Lemon juice for dressing

Prep Time: 15 minutes

Serving Time: 10 minutes

Nutritional Info (per serving):

- Calories: 379
- Protein: 26g
- Omega-3 Fatty Acids: High

- Antioxidants: High

Instructions:

1. In a bowl, combine quinoa, mixed greens, cucumber, and cherry tomatoes.

2. Top with grilled salmon.

3. Drizzle with olive oil and lemon juice.

4. Toss gently and serve.

Serving Methods:

- Garnish with chopped fresh herbs, such as dill or parsley.

- Serve with a side of whole-grain bread.

2. Chickpea and Vegetable Stir-Fry

Ingredients:

- 1 can chickpeas, drained and rinsed

- 1 cup broccoli florets

- 1 bell pepper, sliced

- 1 carrot, julienned

- 2 tablespoons soy sauce

- 1 tablespoon sesame oil

- 1 teaspoon ginger, minced

Prep Time: 15 minutes

Serving Time: 10 minutes

Nutritional Info (per serving):

- Calories: 322

- Protein: 13g

- Fiber: 11g

- Antioxidants: Moderate

Instructions:

1. In a wok or skillet, sauté broccoli, bell pepper, and carrot.

2. Add chickpeas and minced ginger.

3. Drizzle with soy sauce and sesame oil.

4. Stir-fry until vegetables are tender.

5. Serve over brown rice or quinoa.

Serving Methods:

- Sprinkle with sesame seeds for added crunch.

- Top with sliced green onions for extra flavour.

3. Mediterranean Lentil Salad

Ingredients:

- 1 cup cooked lentils

- 1/2 cup cherry tomatoes, halved

- 1/4 cup Kalamata olives, sliced

- 1/4 cup feta cheese, crumbled

- 2 tablespoons olive oil

- 1 tablespoon balsamic vinegar

- Fresh oregano for garnish

Prep Time: 20 minutes

Serving Time: 10 minutes

Nutritional Info (per serving):

- Calories: 359

- Protein: 16g

- Fiber: 10g

- Antioxidants: Moderate

Instructions:

1. Combine cooked lentils, cherry tomatoes, olives, and feta cheese in a bowl.

2. Drizzle with olive oil and balsamic vinegar.

3. Toss gently and garnish with fresh oregano.

4. Serve at room temperature.

Serving Methods:

- Add grilled chicken or tofu for an extra protein boost.

- Serve over a bed of mixed greens for a refreshing twist.

4. Tuna and Avocado Wrap

Ingredients:

- 1 whole-grain wrap

- 1 can tuna, drained

- 1/2 avocado, sliced

- 1/4 cup red onion, thinly sliced

- 1 tablespoon Greek yogurt

- 1 teaspoon Dijon mustard

- Lettuce leaves for wrapping

Prep Time: 10 minutes

Serving Time: 5 minutes

Nutritional Info (per serving):

- Calories: 300

- Protein: 23g

- Omega-3 Fatty Acids: Moderate

Instructions:

1. In a bowl, mix tuna, sliced avocado, red onion, Greek yogurt, and Dijon mustard.

2. Lay out a whole-grain wrap and add lettuce leaves.

3. Spoon the tuna and avocado mixture onto the wrap.

4. Roll up and serve.

Serving Methods:

- Cut into bite-sized pinwheels for a party or snack.

- Serve with a side of vegetable sticks for added crunch.

5. Quinoa and Vegetable Stuffed Bell Peppers

Ingredients:

- 2 bell peppers, halved

- 1 cup cooked quinoa

- 1/2 cup black beans, drained and rinsed

- 1/2 cup corn kernels

- 1/4 cup diced tomatoes

- 1/4 cup shredded cheddar cheese

- 1 teaspoon taco seasoning

Prep Time: 20 minutes

Serving Time: 25 minutes

Nutritional Info (per serving):

- Calories: 281

- Protein: 16g

- Fiber: 9g

- Vitamin C: High

Instructions:

1. Preheat the oven to 375°F (190°C).

2. In a bowl, mix cooked quinoa, black beans, corn, diced tomatoes, taco seasoning, and half of the shredded cheddar cheese.

3. Stuff the bell peppers with the quinoa mixture.

4. Top with the remaining cheddar cheese.

5. Bake until the peppers are tender, about 20-25 minutes.

Serving Methods:

- Drizzle with salsa for extra flavour.

- Serve with a dollop of Greek yogurt on top.

6. Broccoli and Almond Soup

Ingredients:

- 2 cups broccoli florets

- 1 onion, diced

- 2 cloves garlic, minced

- 1/4 cup almonds, chopped

- 4 cups vegetable broth

- 1 tablespoon olive oil

- Salt and pepper to taste

Prep Time: 15 minutes

Serving Time: 25 minutes

Nutritional Info (per serving):

- Calories: 181

- Protein: 9g

- Fiber: 7g

- Vitamin C: High

Instructions:

1. In a pot, sauté onion and garlic in olive oil until softened.

2. Add broccoli, almonds, and vegetable broth.

3. Bring to a boil and simmer until broccoli is tender.

4. Blend the soup until smooth.

5. Season with salt and pepper and serve.

Serving Methods:

- Garnish with a sprinkle of chopped almonds.

- Serve with a side of whole-grain bread.

7. Grilled Chicken and Quinoa Bowl

Ingredients:

- 1 cup cooked quinoa

- 4 oz grilled chicken breast, sliced

- 1 cup mixed vegetables (bell peppers, zucchini, cherry tomatoes)

- 1 tablespoon olive oil

- 1 tablespoon balsamic vinegar

- Fresh basil for garnish

Prep Time: 15 minutes

Serving Time: 10 minutes

Nutritional Info (per serving):

- Calories: 300

- Protein: 27g

- Fiber: 9g

- Antioxidants: Moderate

Instructions:

1. In a bowl, combine cooked quinoa, grilled chicken, and mixed vegetables.

2. Drizzle with olive oil and balsamic vinegar.

3. Toss gently and garnish with fresh basil.

4. Serve warm or at room temperature.

Serving Methods:

- Top with crumbled feta cheese for added richness.

- Serve over a bed of spinach or arugula.

8. Vegetarian Lentil and Spinach Curry

Ingredients:

- 1 cup cooked lentils

- 2 cups spinach leaves

- 1 onion, diced

- 2 tomatoes, chopped

- 1 tablespoon curry powder

- 1/2 teaspoon turmeric

- 1/2 cup coconut milk

- 1 tablespoon olive oil

Prep Time: 20 minutes

Serving Time: 25 minutes

Nutritional Info (per serving):

- Calories: 288

- Protein: 17g

- Fiber: 15g

- Anti-Inflammatory Compounds: High

Instructions:

1. In a pan, sauté diced onion in olive oil until translucent.

2. Add chopped tomatoes, curry powder, and turmeric.

3. Stir in cooked lentils and spinach.

4. Pour in coconut milk and simmer until spinach wilts.

5. Serve over brown rice or quinoa.

Serving Methods:

- Garnish with chopped cilantro for freshness.

- Serve with a side of whole-grain naan bread.

9. Greek Salad with Grilled Shrimp

Ingredients:

- 1 cup mixed greens

- 8 large shrimp, grilled

- 1/2 cup cherry tomatoes, halved

- 1/4 cup cucumber, sliced

- 1/4 cup feta cheese, crumbled

- 1/4 cup Kalamata olives, sliced

- Greek dressing (olive oil, lemon juice, oregano)

Prep Time: 15 minutes

Serving Time: 10 minutes

Nutritional Info (per serving):

- Calories: 300

- Protein: 25g

- Antioxidants: Moderate

Instructions:

1. Arrange mixed greens on a plate.

2. Top with grilled shrimp, cherry tomatoes, cucumber, feta cheese, and olives.

3. Drizzle with Greek dressing.

4. Serve chilled.

Serving Methods:

- Sprinkle with pine nuts for added crunch.

- Serve with a side of whole-grain pita bread.

10. Tomato Basil Quinoa Soup

Ingredients:

- 1 cup cooked quinoa

- 2 cups tomatoes, diced

- 1/2 cup carrots, diced

- 1/2 onion, diced

- 2 cloves garlic, minced

- 1 cup vegetable broth

- Fresh basil leaves for garnish

- Salt and pepper to taste

Prep Time: 20 minutes

Serving Time: 25 minutes

Nutritional Info (per serving):

- Calories: 222

- Protein: 9g

- Vitamin C: High

- Anti-Inflammatory Compounds: Moderate

Instructions:

1. Sauté diced onion and minced garlic until softened.

2. Add diced tomatoes, carrots, and vegetable broth.

3. Simmer until vegetables are tender.

4. Stir in cooked quinoa.

5. Season with salt and pepper, garnish with fresh basil, and serve.

Serving Methods:

- Top with a dollop of Greek yogurt for creaminess.

- Serve with a side of whole-grain crackers.

Dinner Recipes

These ten (10) dinner dishes for a cancer-fighting diet include all the necessary ingredients, preparation and serving times, nutritional data, recipe notes, and two ways to present the dish.

1. Grilled Salmon with Quinoa and Roasted Vegetables

Ingredients:

- 6 oz salmon fillet

- 1 cup cooked quinoa

- 1 cup mixed vegetables (zucchini, bell peppers, cherry tomatoes)

- 1 tablespoon olive oil

- Lemon wedges for garnish

- Fresh dill for garnish

Prep Time: 20 minutes

Serving Time: 15 minutes

Nutritional Info (per serving):

- Calories: 400

- Protein: 29g

- Omega-3 Fatty Acids: High

- Antioxidants: High

Instructions:

1. Season the salmon fillet with salt and pepper.

2. Grill the salmon until cooked through.

3. In a separate pan, roast mixed vegetables in olive oil.

4. Serve grilled salmon on a bed of cooked quinoa, surrounded by roasted vegetables.

5. Garnish with lemon wedges and fresh dill.

Serving Methods:

- Drizzle with a balsamic glaze for added flavour.

- Serve with a side of steamed asparagus.

2. Vegetarian Stir-Fried Tofu with Broccoli and Brown Rice

Ingredients:

- 8 oz firm tofu, cubed

- 1 cup broccoli florets

- 1 bell pepper, sliced

- 1 cup snap peas

- 2 tablespoons soy sauce

- 1 tablespoon sesame oil

- 1 teaspoon ginger, minced

Prep Time: 20 minutes

Cooking Time: 15 minutes

Nutritional Info (per serving):

- Calories: 400

- Protein: 23g

- Fiber: 9g

- Antioxidants: Moderate

Instructions:

1. Press tofu to remove excess water, then cube it.

2. Sauté tofu until golden brown.

3. Add broccoli, bell pepper, snap peas, and minced ginger.

4. Stir in soy sauce and sesame oil.

5. Serve over brown rice.

Serving Methods:

- Sprinkle with sesame seeds for added crunch.

- Top with sliced green onions for extra flavour.

3. Mushroom and Spinach Stuffed Chicken Breast

Ingredients:

- 2 boneless, skinless chicken breasts
- 1 cup mushrooms, finely chopped
- 1 cup spinach, chopped
- 1/4 cup feta cheese, crumbled
- 1 tablespoon olive oil
- Salt and pepper to taste
- Lemon wedges for garnish

Prep Time: 25 minutes

Serving Time: 25 minutes

Nutritional Info (per serving):

- Calories: 320
- Protein: 44g
- Vitamin D: Moderate
- Antioxidants: Moderate

Instructions:

1. Preheat the oven to 375°F (190°C).

2. In a pan, sauté mushrooms and spinach in olive oil until cooked.

3. Butterfly the chicken breasts and stuff with the mushroom and spinach mixture.

4. Season with salt and pepper.

5. Bake until the chicken is cooked through.

6. Garnish with lemon wedges and serve.

Serving Methods:

- Drizzle with a balsamic reduction for added sweetness.

- Serve with a side of quinoa.

4. Lentil and Vegetable Curry

Ingredients:

- 1 cup dry lentils, cooked

- 1 cup broccoli, chopped

- 1 cup cauliflower, chopped

- 1 cup carrots, sliced

- 1 onion, diced

- 2 cloves garlic, minced

- 1 can (14 oz) coconut milk

- 2 tablespoons curry powder

Prep Time: 25 minutes

Serving Time: 30 minutes

Nutritional Info (per serving):

- Calories: 329

- Protein: 16g

- Fiber: 15g

- Anti-Inflammatory Compounds: High

Instructions:

1. In a pot, sauté onions and garlic until softened.

2. Add curry powder and stir.

3. Add cooked lentils, broccoli, cauliflower, carrots, and coconut milk.

4. Simmer until vegetables are tender.

5. Serve over brown rice.

Serving Methods:

- Garnish with fresh cilantro for added freshness.

- Serve with a side of whole-grain naan bread.

5. Baked Cod with Quinoa and Roasted Brussels Sprouts

Ingredients:

- 6 oz cod fillet

- 1 cup cooked quinoa

- 1 cup Brussels sprouts, halved

- 1 tablespoon olive oil

- Lemon wedges for garnish

- Fresh parsley for garnish

Prep Time: 20 minutes

Serving Time: 20 minutes

Nutritional Info (per serving):

- Calories: 356

- Protein: 26g

- Omega-3 Fatty Acids: High

- Vitamin C: High

Instructions:

1. Preheat the oven to 400°F (200°C).

2. Toss Brussels sprouts in olive oil and roast until golden brown.

3. Season cod fillet with salt and pepper.

4. Bake cod in the oven until cooked through.

5. Serve cod on a bed of quinoa, surrounded by roasted Brussels sprouts.

6. Garnish with lemon wedges and fresh parsley.

Serving Methods:

- Drizzle with a garlic and herb sauce for added flavour.

- Serve with a side of steamed green beans.

6. Spaghetti Squash with Tomato and Basil Sauce

Ingredients:

- 1 spaghetti squash, halved and seeded

- 2 cups cherry tomatoes, halved

- 2 cloves garlic, minced

- 1/4 cup fresh basil, chopped

- 1 tablespoon olive oil

- 1/4 cup Parmesan cheese, grated

Prep Time: 15 minutes

Serving Time: 45 minutes

Nutritional Info (per serving):

- Calories: 220

- Protein: 5g

- Fiber: 8g

- Vitamin C: High

Instructions:

1. Preheat the oven to 375°F (190°C).

2. Brush spaghetti squash halves with olive oil and roast until tender.

3. In a pan, sauté garlic until fragrant.

4. Add cherry tomatoes and cook until softened.

5. Scrape the spaghetti squash strands into the pan and mix.

6. Stir in fresh basil and top with Parmesan cheese.

Serving Methods:

- Top with pine nuts for added texture.

- Serve with a side of mixed greens.

7. Turkey and Vegetable Skewers with Quinoa

Ingredients:

- 8 oz turkey breast, cubed

- 1 bell pepper, cut into chunks

- 1 zucchini, sliced

- 1 cup cherry tomatoes

- 1 cup cooked quinoa

- 2 tablespoons olive oil

- 1 teaspoon smoked paprika

- Salt and pepper to taste

Prep Time: 25 minutes

Serving Time: 15 minutes

Nutritional Info (per serving):

- Calories: 340

- Protein: 28g

- Fiber: 8g

- Antioxidants: Moderate

Instructions:

1. Preheat the grill or oven to medium-high heat.

2. Thread turkey, bell pepper, zucchini, and cherry tomatoes onto skewers.

3. Mix olive oil, smoked paprika, salt, and pepper in a bowl.

4. Brush skewers with the oil mixture and grill until turkey is cooked.

5. Serve over a bed of cooked quinoa.

Serving Methods:

- Drizzle with a squeeze of lemon for brightness.

- Serve with a side of tzatziki sauce.

8. Cauliflower and Chickpea Curry

Ingredients:

- 1 cup cauliflower florets

- 1 can chickpeas, drained and rinsed

- 1 onion, diced

- 2 cloves garlic, minced

- 1 can (14 oz) diced tomatoes

- 1/2 cup coconut milk

- 1 tablespoon curry powder

Prep Time: 20 minutes

Serving Time: 25 minutes

Nutritional Info (per serving):

- Calories: 280

- Protein: 12g

- Fiber: 10g

- Anti-Inflammatory Compounds: High

Instructions:

1. Sauté onions and garlic in a pan until softened.

2. Add cauliflower, chickpeas, diced tomatoes, coconut milk, and curry powder.

3. Simmer until cauliflower is tender.

4. Serve over quinoa or brown rice.

Serving Methods:

- Garnish with chopped cilantro for freshness.

- Serve with a side of whole-grain pita bread.

9. Baked Sweet Potato and Black Bean Enchiladas

Ingredients:

- 2 large sweet potatoes, roasted and mashed

- 1 can black beans, drained and rinsed

- 1 cup corn kernels

- 1 cup spinach, chopped

- 8 whole-grain tortillas

- 1 cup enchilada sauce

- 1/2 cup shredded cheddar cheese

Prep Time: 30 minutes

Serving Time: 25 minutes

Nutritional Info (per serving):

- Calories: 300

- Protein: 15g

- Fiber: 12g

- Vitamin A: High

Instructions:

1. Preheat the oven to 375°F (190°C).

2. In a bowl, mix mashed sweet potatoes, black beans, corn, and spinach.

3. Spoon the mixture onto tortillas and roll them up.

4. Place the enchiladas in a baking dish, cover with enchilada sauce, and sprinkle with cheddar cheese.

5. Bake until cheese is melted and bubbly.

Serving Methods:

- Top with a dollop of Greek yogurt for creaminess.

- Serve with a side of avocado slices.

10. Quinoa and Kale Stuffed Bell Peppers

Ingredients:

- 4 bell peppers, halved and seeded

- 1 cup cooked quinoa

- 1 cup kale, chopped

- 1 can (14 oz) diced tomatoes

- 1 cup black beans, drained and rinsed

- 1 teaspoon cumin

- 1/2 teaspoon chili powder

Prep Time: 20 minutes

Serving Time: 30 minutes

Nutritional Info (per serving):

- Calories: 300

- Protein: 16g

- Fiber: 12g

- Vitamin C: High

Instructions:

1. Preheat the oven to 375°F (190°C).

2. In a bowl, mix cooked quinoa, chopped kale, diced tomatoes, black beans, cumin, and chili powder.

3. Stuff bell peppers with the quinoa mixture.

4. Bake until peppers are tender.

Serving Methods:

- Top with a dollop of salsa for added flavour.

- Serve with a side of mixed greens.

Snacks Recipes

The following list of ten cancer-fighting snack recipes includes information on ingredients, preparation and serving times, nutritional value, and two ways to serve.

1. Hummus and Veggie Sticks

Ingredients:

- 1 cup chickpeas, drained

- 2 tablespoons tahini

- 2 tablespoons olive oil

- 1 clove garlic, minced

- Juice of 1 lemon

- Carrot and cucumber stick for dipping

Prep Time: 10 minutes

Serving Time: 5 minutes

Nutritional Info (per serving):

- Calories: 150

- Protein: 5g

- Fiber: 6g

- Antioxidants: Moderate

Instructions:

1. Blend chickpeas, tahini, olive oil, garlic, and lemon juice until smooth.

2. Serve hummus with carrot and cucumber sticks for dipping.

Serving Methods:

- Sprinkle with paprika or cumin for added flavour.

- Garnish with chopped parsley or cilantro.

2. Greek Yogurt Parfait with Berries

Ingredients:

- 1 cup Greek yogurt

- 1/2 cup mixed berries (blueberries, strawberries, raspberries)

- 2 tablespoons granola

- 1 tablespoon honey

Prep Time: 5 minutes

Serving Time: 5 minutes

Nutritional Info (per serving):

- Calories: 200

- Protein: 14g

- Antioxidants: High

Instructions:

1. Layer Greek yogurt, mixed berries, and granola in a glass.

2. Drizzle with honey before serving.

Serving Methods:

- Top with a sprinkle of chia seeds for added nutrition.

- Serve in a bowl for a quick and easy snack.

3. Avocado and Tomato Salsa with Whole-Grain Crackers

Ingredients:

- 1 ripe avocado, diced

- 1 cup cherry tomatoes, diced

- 1/4 cup red onion, finely chopped

- 1/4 cup cilantro, chopped

- Whole-grain crackers for serving

Prep Time: 10 minutes

Serving Time: 5 minutes

Nutritional Info (per serving):

- Calories: 184

- Fiber: 6g

- Vitamin C: High

- Anti-Inflammatory Compounds: Moderate

Instructions:

1. Mix diced avocado, cherry tomatoes, red onion, and cilantro in a bowl.

2. Serve with whole-grain crackers for dipping.

Serving Methods:

- Squeeze fresh lime juice over the salsa for extra zing.

- Garnish with a dash of black pepper.

4. Almond Butter and Banana Toast

Ingredients:

- 2 slices whole-grain bread

- 2 tablespoons almond butter

- 1 banana, sliced

- Chia seeds for sprinkling

Prep Time: 5 minutes

Serving Time: 5 minutes

Nutritional Info (per serving):

- Calories: 283

- Protein: 12g

- Fiber: 8g

- Omega-3 Fatty Acids: Moderate

Instructions:

1. Toast whole-grain bread slices.

2. Spread almond butter on the toast.

3.   Top with banana slices and sprinkle with chia seeds.

Serving Methods:

- Drizzle with honey for added sweetness.

- Serve with a side of mixed berries.

5. Cucumber and Hummus Bites

Ingredients:

- 1 cucumber, sliced into rounds

- 1/2 cup hummus

- Cherry tomatoes for topping

- Fresh basil leaves for garnish

Prep Time: 10 minutes

Serving Time: 5 minutes

Nutritional Info (per serving):

- Calories: 120

- Protein: 5g

- Fiber: 4g

- Antioxidants: Moderate

Instructions:

1.   Top cucumber rounds with a dollop of hummus.

2. Place a cherry tomato on each and garnish with fresh basil.

Serving Methods:

- Sprinkle with a pinch of sea salt for enhanced flavor.

- Serve on a platter for a stylish presentation.

6. Quinoa and Edamame Salad Cups

Ingredients:

- 1 cup cooked quinoa

- 1/2 cup edamame, shelled

- 1/4 cup red bell pepper, diced

- 1/4 cup cucumber, diced

- 2 tablespoons balsamic vinaigrette

- Endive or lettuce leaves for serving

Prep Time: 15 minutes

Serving Time: 10 minutes

Nutritional Info (per serving):

- Calories: 184

- Protein: 10g

- Fiber: 7g

- Antioxidants: High

Instructions:

1. In a bowl, combine quinoa, edamame, red bell pepper, and cucumber.

2. Drizzle with balsamic vinaigrette and toss.

3. Spoon the mixture into endive or lettuce leaves.

Serving Methods:

- Top with crumbled feta cheese for added richness.

- Serve as an elegant appetizer at gatherings.

7. Sliced Apple with Nut Butter

Ingredients:

- 1 apple, sliced

- 2 tablespoons nut butter (almond, peanut, or cashew)

- Cinnamon for sprinkling

Prep Time: 5 minutes

Serving Time: 5 minutes

Nutritional Info (per serving):

- Calories: 227

- Protein: 7g

- Fiber: 8g

- Antioxidants: Moderate

Instructions:

1. Arrange apple slices on a plate.

2. Spread nut butter on each slice.

3. Sprinkle with cinnamon before serving.

Serving Methods:

- Top with a handful of walnuts or almonds for crunch.

- Serve with a side of low-fat yogurt.

8. Kale Chips with Parmesan

Ingredients:

- 2 cups kale, torn into bite-sized pieces

- 1 tablespoon olive oil

- 2 tablespoons Parmesan cheese, grated

- Sea salt for sprinkling

Prep Time: 10 minutes

Serving Time: 15 minutes

Nutritional Info (per serving):

- Calories: 129

- Protein: 7g

- Vitamin A and K: High

Instructions:

1. Preheat the oven to 350°F (175°C).

2. Toss kale with olive oil and spread on a baking sheet.

3. Sprinkle with Parmesan and sea salt.

4. Bake until crispy, about 15 minutes.

Serving Methods:

- Squeeze fresh lemon juice over the chips for brightness.

- Serve in a bowl as a crunchy alternative to potato chips.

9. Chia Seed Pudding with Mango

Ingredients:

- 2 tablespoons chia seeds

- 1/2 cup almond milk

- 1/2 teaspoon vanilla extract

- 1/2 cup diced mango

- 1 tablespoon shredded coconut

Prep Time: 5 minutes (+overnight chilling)

Serving Time: 5 minutes

Nutritional Info (per serving):

- Calories: 189

- Fiber: 9g

- Omega-3 Fatty Acids: Moderate

Instructions:

1. Mix chia seeds, almond milk, and vanilla extract in a jar.

2. Refrigerate overnight.

3. Top with diced mango and shredded coconut before serving.

Serving Methods:

- Drizzle with honey or maple syrup for sweetness.

- Serve in small jars for a portable snack.

10. Trail Mix with Nuts and Dried Berries

Ingredients:

- 1/2 cup mixed nuts (almonds, walnuts, cashews)

- 1/4 cup dried berries (blueberries, cranberries)

- 2 tablespoons dark chocolate chips

- Pumpkin seeds for crunch

Prep Time: 5 minutes

Serving Time: 5 minutes

Nutritional Info (per serving):

- Calories: 279

- Protein: 9g

- Antioxidants: Moderate

Instructions:

1. Mix nuts, dried berries, dark chocolate chips, and pumpkin seeds in a bowl.

2. Portion into snack-sized servings.

Serving Methods:

- Divide into small bags for an on-the-go snack.

- Sprinkle with a pinch of sea salt for flavour.

Desserts Recipes

Listed below are ten dessert recipes from the cancer-fighting diet, together with information on ingredients, preparation and serving times, nutritional value, and two ways to serve.

1. Berry and Yogurt Parfait

Ingredients:

- 1 cup mixed berries (strawberries, blueberries, raspberries)
- 1 cup Greek yogurt
- 2 tablespoons honey
- 1/4 cup granola

Prep Time: 10 minutes

Serving Time: 5 minutes

Nutritional Info (per serving):

- Calories: 189
- Protein: 14g
- Antioxidants: High

Instructions:

1. Layer Greek yogurt at the bottom of a glass or bowl.
2. Add mixed berries on top.

3. Drizzle with honey.

4. Repeat the layers.

5. Sprinkle granola on the top layer.

Serving Methods:

- Garnish with mint leaves for freshness.

- Serve with a side of dark chocolate shavings.

2. Avocado Chocolate Mousse

Ingredients:

- 2 ripe avocados

- 1/4 cup cocoa powder

- 1/4 cup maple syrup

- 1 teaspoon vanilla extract

- A pinch of sea salt

Prep Time: 15 minutes

Serving Time: 2 hours (chilled)

Nutritional Info (per serving):

- Calories: 300

- Healthy Fats: High

- Antioxidants: Moderate

Instructions:

1. Blend avocados, cocoa powder, maple syrup, vanilla extract, and salt until smooth.

2. Chill the mixture in the refrigerator for at least 2 hours.

3. Serve in small bowls or glasses.

Serving Methods:

- Top with sliced strawberries for extra flavor.

- Serve with a sprinkle of crushed nuts.

3. Chia Seed Pudding with Mango and Coconut

Ingredients:

- 3 tablespoons chia seeds

- 1 cup almond milk

- 1/2 teaspoon vanilla extract

- 1/2 cup diced mango

- 2 tablespoons shredded coconut

Prep Time: 5 minutes (+overnight chilling)

Serving Time: 5 minutes

Nutritional Info (per serving):

- Calories: 200

- Fiber: 9g

- Omega-3 Fatty Acids: Moderate

Instructions:

1. Mix chia seeds, almond milk, and vanilla extract in a jar.

2. Refrigerate overnight or for at least 4 hours.

3. Layer with diced mango and shredded coconut before serving.

Serving Methods:

- Drizzle with a bit of honey for sweetness.

- Serve with a dollop of Greek yogurt on top.

4. Baked Apples with Cinnamon and Walnuts

Ingredients:

- 2 apples, cored and halved

- 1 teaspoon cinnamon

- 1/4 cup chopped walnuts

- 1 tablespoon honey

Prep Time: 10 minutes

Serving Time: 5 minutes

Nutritional Info (per serving):

- Calories: 150

- Fiber: 5g

- Antioxidants: Moderate

Instructions:

1. Preheat the oven to 375°F (190°C).

2. Place apples in a baking dish.

3. Sprinkle with cinnamon and chopped walnuts.

4. Drizzle honey over the top.

5. Bake until apples are tender, about 20 minutes.

Serving Methods:

- Top with a scoop of vanilla yogurt.

- Serve with a sprinkle of ground flaxseeds.

5. Dark Chocolate and Berry Bark

Ingredients:

- 1 cup dark chocolate (70% cocoa or higher)

- 1/2 cup mixed berries (strawberries, blueberries, raspberries)

- 2 tablespoons chopped nuts (almonds, walnuts)

Prep Time: 15 minutes

Serving Time: 1 hour (chilled)

Nutritional Info (per serving):

- Calories: 170

- Antioxidants: High

Instructions:

1. Melt dark chocolate in a heatproof bowl.

2. Line a baking sheet with parchment paper.

3. Pour melted chocolate onto the parchment paper.

4. Sprinkle mixed berries and chopped nuts over the chocolate.

5. Chill in the refrigerator for at least 1 hour.

6. Break into pieces before serving.

Serving Methods:

- Serve with a side of fresh berries.

- Garnish with a sprinkle of sea salt.

6. Cinnamon Baked Pears with Greek Yogurt

Ingredients:

- 2 ripe pears, halved and cored

- 1 teaspoon cinnamon

- 2 tablespoons chopped almonds

- 1/4 cup Greek yogurt

Prep Time: 10 minutes

Serving Time: 5 minutes

Nutritional Info (per serving):

- Calories: 170

- Protein: 6g

- Fiber: 8g

Instructions:

1. Preheat the oven to 375°F (190°C).

2. Place pear halves in a baking dish.

3. Sprinkle with cinnamon and chopped almonds.

4. Bake until pears are tender, about 20 minutes.

5. Serve with a dollop of Greek yogurt.

Serving Methods:

- Drizzle with a touch of honey for sweetness.

- Serve with a sprinkle of ground flaxseeds.

7. Coconut and Berry Popsicles

Ingredients:

- 1 cup mixed berries (strawberries, blueberries, raspberries)
- 1 can (14 oz) coconut milk
- 2 tablespoons honey
- 1 teaspoon vanilla extract

Prep Time: 10 minutes (+freezing time)

Serving Time: 5 minutes

Nutritional Info (per serving):

- Calories: 120
- Antioxidants: High

Instructions:

1. Blend mixed berries, coconut milk, honey, and vanilla extract until smooth.

2. Pour the mixture into popsicle molds.

3. Freeze until solid, at least 4 hours.

4. Run molds under warm water to release popsicles.

Serving Methods:

- Roll popsicles in shredded coconut before serving.

- Serve with a side of fresh berries.

8. Turmeric and Ginger Golden Milk Popsicles

Ingredients:

- 1 can (14 oz) coconut milk

- 1 teaspoon turmeric powder

- 1/2 teaspoon ginger, grated

- 2 tablespoons honey

- A pinch of black pepper

Prep Time: 10 minutes (+freezing time)

Serving Time: 5 minutes

Nutritional Info (per serving):

- Calories: 153

- Anti-Inflammatory Compounds: High

Instructions:

1. Whisk together coconut milk, turmeric, ginger, honey, and black pepper.

2. Pour the mixture into popsicle molds.

3. Freeze until solid, at least 4 hours.

4. Run molds under warm water to release popsicles.

Serving Methods:

- Sprinkle with chopped pistachios for added texture.

- Serve with a side of fresh pineapple.

9. Pomegranate and Pistachio Yogurt Parfait

Ingredients:

- 1 cup Greek yogurt

- 1/2 cup pomegranate seeds

- 2 tablespoons chopped pistachios

- 1 tablespoon honey

Prep Time: 10 minutes

Serving Time: 5 minutes

Nutritional Info (per serving):

- Calories: 232

- Protein: 16g

- Antioxidants: High

Instructions:

1. In a glass or bowl, layer Greek yogurt, pomegranate seeds, and chopped pistachios.

2. Drizzle with honey before serving.

Serving Methods:

- Top with a sprinkle of ground flaxseeds.

- Serve with a side of dark chocolate.

10. Frozen Banana Bites

Ingredients:

- 2 bananas, sliced

- 1/4 cup almond butter

- 1/4 cup dark chocolate (70% cocoa or higher)

- 2 tablespoons shredded coconut

Prep Time: 15 minutes (+freezing time)

Serving Time: 5 minutes

Nutritional Info (per serving):

- Calories: 168

- Healthy Fats: High

- Antioxidants: Moderate

Instructions:

1. Spread almond butter on banana slices and sandwich them together.

2. Freeze banana bites until solid, about 2 hours.

3. Melt dark chocolate in a heatproof bowl.

4. Dip frozen banana bites in melted chocolate and sprinkle with shredded coconut.

5. Freeze again until chocolate is set.

Serving Methods:

- Serve with a side of mixed berries.

- Drizzle with a touch of honey before serving.

21 Days Meal Plan

These recipes for breakfast, lunch, dinner, and desserts, along with some of the dessert selections, are included in this 21-day cancer-fighting diet plan. Per your specific dietary requirements, feel free to modify the serving sizes and amounts.

Week 1:

Day 1:

- **Breakfast:** Avocado Toast with Poached Eggs

- **Lunch:** Quinoa Salad with Chickpeas and Veggies

- **Dinner:** Grilled Salmon with Quinoa and Roasted Vegetables

- **Dessert:** Berry and Yogurt Parfait

Day 2:

- **Breakfast:** Greek Yogurt Smoothie with Berries and Spinach

- **Lunch:** Lentil and Vegetable Curry

- **Dinner:** Vegetarian Stir-Fried Tofu with Broccoli and Brown Rice

- **Dessert:** Avocado Chocolate Mousse

Day 3:

- **Breakfast:** Overnight Oats with Chia Seeds and Mixed Berries

- **Lunch:** Baked Sweet Potato and Black Bean Enchiladas

- **Dinner:** Mushroom and Spinach Stuffed Chicken Breast

- **Dessert:** Chia Seed Pudding with Mango and Coconut

Day 4:

- **Breakfast:** Whole Grain Pancakes with Fresh Berries

- **Lunch:** Turkey and Vegetable Skewers with Quinoa

- **Dinner:** Baked Cod with Quinoa and Roasted Brussels Sprouts

- **Dessert:** Baked Apples with Cinnamon and Walnuts

Day 5:

- **Breakfast:** Vegetable Omelette with Whole Grain Toast

- **Lunch:** Greek Salad with Grilled Shrimp

- **Dinner:** Cauliflower and Chickpea Curry

- **Dessert:** Dark Chocolate and Berry Bark

Day 6:

- **Breakfast:** Spinach and Feta Breakfast Wrap

- **Lunch:** Greek Quinoa Salad with Feta and Olives

- **Dinner:** Spaghetti Squash with Tomato and Basil Sauce

- **Dessert:** Cinnamon Baked Pears with Greek Yogurt

Day 7:

- **Breakfast:** Mixed Berry Smoothie Bowl with Granola

- **Lunch:** Quinoa and Kale Stuffed Bell Peppers

- **Dinner:** Lentil and Spinach Soup with Whole Grain Crackers

- **Dessert:** Coconut and Berry Popsicles

Week 2:

Day 8:

- **Breakfast:** Avocado Toast with Poached Eggs

- **Lunch:** Quinoa Salad with Chickpeas and Veggies

- **Dinner:** Grilled Salmon with Quinoa and Roasted Vegetables

- **Dessert:** Berry and Yogurt Parfait

Day 9:

- **Breakfast:** Greek Yogurt Smoothie with Berries and Spinach

- **Lunch:** Lentil and Vegetable Curry

- **Dinner:** Vegetarian Stir-Fried Tofu with Broccoli and Brown Rice

- **Dessert:** Avocado Chocolate Mousse

Day 10:

- **Breakfast:** Overnight Oats with Chia Seeds and Mixed Berries

- **Lunch:** Baked Sweet Potato and Black Bean Enchiladas

- **Dinner:** Mushroom and Spinach Stuffed Chicken Breast

- **Dessert:** Chia Seed Pudding with Mango and Coconut

Day 11:

- **Breakfast:** Whole Grain Pancakes with Fresh Berries

- **Lunch:** Turkey and Vegetable Skewers with Quinoa

- **Dinner:** Baked Cod with Quinoa and Roasted Brussels Sprouts

- **Dessert:** Baked Apples with Cinnamon and Walnuts

Day 12:

- **Breakfast:** Vegetable Omelette with Whole Grain Toast

- **Lunch:** Greek Salad with Grilled Shrimp

- **Dinner:** Cauliflower and Chickpea Curry

- **Dessert:** Dark Chocolate and Berry Bark

Day 13:

- **Breakfast:** Spinach and Feta Breakfast Wrap

- **Lunch:** Greek Quinoa Salad with Feta and Olives

- **Dinner:** Spaghetti Squash with Tomato and Basil Sauce

- **Dessert:** Cinnamon Baked Pears with Greek Yogurt

Day 14:

- **Breakfast:** Mixed Berry Smoothie Bowl with Granola

- **Lunch:** Quinoa and Kale Stuffed Bell Peppers

- **Dinner:** Lentil and Spinach Soup with Whole Grain Crackers

- **Dessert:** Coconut and Berry Popsicles

Week 3:

Day 15:

- **Breakfast:** Avocado Toast with Poached Eggs

- **Lunch:** Quinoa Salad with Chickpeas and Veggies

- **Dinner:** Grilled Salmon with Quinoa and Roasted Vegetables

- **Dessert:** Berry and Yogurt Parfait

Day 16:

- **Breakfast:** Greek Yogurt Smoothie with Berries and Spinach

- **Lunch:** Lentil and Vegetable Curry

- **Dinner:** Vegetarian Stir-Fried Tofu with Broccoli and Brown Rice

- **Dessert:** Avocado Chocolate Mousse

Day 17:

- **Breakfast:** Overnight Oats with Chia Seeds and Mixed Berries

- **Lunch:** Baked Sweet Potato and Black Bean Enchiladas

- **Dinner:** Mushroom and Spinach Stuffed Chicken Breast

- **Dessert:** Chia Seed Pudding with Mango and Coconut

Day 18:

- **Breakfast:** Whole Grain Pancakes with Fresh Berries

- **Lunch:** Turkey and Vegetable Skewers with Quinoa

- **Dinner:** Baked Cod with Quinoa and Roasted Brussels Sprouts

- **Dessert:** Baked Apples with Cinnamon and Walnuts

Day 19:

- **Breakfast:** Vegetable Omelette with Whole Grain Toast

- **Lunch:** Greek Salad with Grilled Shrimp

- **Dinner:** Cauliflower and Chickpea Curry

- **Dessert:** Dark Chocolate and Berry Bark

Day 20:

- **Breakfast:** Spinach and Feta Breakfast Wrap

- **Lunch:** Greek Quinoa Salad with Feta and Olives

- **Dinner:** Spaghetti Squash with Tomato and Basil Sauce

- **Dessert:** Cinnamon Baked Pears with Greek Yogurt

Day 21:

- **Breakfast:** Mixed Berry Smoothie Bowl with Granola

- **Lunch:** Quinoa and Kale Stuffed Bell Peppers

- **Dinner:** Lentil and Spinach Soup with Whole Grain Crackers

- **Dessert:** Coconut and Berry Popsicles

CHAPTER SIX

FITNESS AND ITS SYNERGY WITH NUTRITION

The Role of Exercise in Cancer Prevention

Exercise is essential for preserving general health and wellbeing, and its importance in preventing cancer cannot be emphasized. Regular exercise has been linked to a host of health advantages, and an increasing body of research indicates a direct association between physical activity and a lower risk of cancer. We will thoroughly examine the various ways that exercise helps prevent cancer in this discussion, keeping in mind the significance of providing information that is both pertinent and understandable to people.

1. Reducing the Risk of Several Cancer Types:

- Numerous studies have demonstrated a consistent link between regular exercise and a decreased risk of developing various types of cancers, including breast, colorectal, prostate, and lung cancers. Engaging in physical activity is associated with a lower incidence of these cancers, providing a compelling incentive for individuals to incorporate exercise into their daily lives.

2. Modulating Hormone Levels:

- Exercise has the capacity to influence hormonal levels in the body, particularly sex hormones such as estrogen and testosterone. Hormonal imbalances have been implicated in the development of certain cancers, and regular physical activity helps regulate these hormones, thereby reducing the likelihood of cancer initiation and progression.

3. Enhancing Immune Function:

- A robust immune system is instrumental in recognizing and eliminating abnormal cells, including those that could potentially become cancerous. Regular exercise has been shown to enhance immune function, improving the body's ability to detect and eradicate cancer cells before they can develop into a full-fledged malignancy.

4. Managing Body Weight:

- Maintaining a healthy body weight is a key aspect of cancer prevention, as obesity is a known risk factor for several types of cancer. Exercise aids in weight management by promoting calorie expenditure and optimizing metabolism. Individuals who engage in regular physical activity are more likely to achieve and sustain a healthy weight, consequently reducing their risk of obesity-related cancers.

5. Improving Insulin Sensitivity:

- Insulin resistance and elevated insulin levels are factors associated with an increased risk of certain cancers, including colorectal and pancreatic cancers. Exercise improves insulin sensitivity, helping to regulate blood sugar levels and mitigate these risk factors, thereby contributing to cancer prevention.

6. Facilitating Bowel Regularity:

- Regular physical activity has a positive impact on gastrointestinal health by promoting bowel regularity. Adequate bowel function is associated with a decreased risk of colorectal cancer, making exercise an essential lifestyle factor in preventing malignancies of the digestive system.

7. Reducing Chronic Inflammation:

- Chronic inflammation is a common denominator in many chronic diseases, including cancer. Regular exercise has anti-inflammatory effects, helping to mitigate the systemic inflammation that may contribute to the development and progression of cancer.

8. Enhancing Mental Health:

- Exercise is not only beneficial for physical health but also plays a crucial role in promoting mental well-being. Mental health is intricately connected to overall health, and a positive mindset facilitated by regular exercise may contribute to a reduced risk of certain cancers.

Tailoring Fitness Routines for Cancer Patients

Maintaining a fitness regimen both during and after cancer treatment calls for careful planning and customized strategy. Given the particular difficulties faced by cancer patients, a customized exercise program can be quite beneficial for enhancing both physical and emotional health. In order to make the information relevant and useful to people, we will thoroughly examine the factors and techniques that go into creating exercise regimens especially for those receiving or recovering from cancer treatment in this talk.

1. Understanding Individual Health Status:

- Each cancer patient is unique, and their fitness plan should reflect their individual health status. Factors such as the type of cancer, stage of treatment, and any pre-existing health conditions must be considered.

Collaborating with healthcare professionals, including oncologists and physical therapists, is essential to gather insights into the patient's health and determine appropriate starting points for exercise.

2. Incorporating Aerobic Exercise:

- Aerobic exercise, such as walking, cycling, or swimming, can be beneficial for cancer patients. It helps improve cardiovascular health, boost energy levels, and enhance mood. The intensity and duration of aerobic activities should be gradually increased based on the patient's tolerance and response to treatment.

3. Implementing Strength Training:

- Strength training is vital for maintaining muscle mass and bone density, especially as cancer treatments may contribute to muscle loss. Tailored strength training exercises, using body weight, resistance bands, or light weights, can be incorporated to improve overall strength and functionality.

4. Prioritizing Flexibility and Range of Motion:

- Cancer treatments and the associated sedentary periods can lead to reduced flexibility and joint mobility. Including gentle stretching exercises and activities that focus on improving range of motion helps enhance flexibility, reduce stiffness, and maintain joint health.

5. Addressing Fatigue and Energy Conservation:

- Cancer-related fatigue is a common challenge for patients. Fitness routines should be designed to address fatigue while promoting energy conservation. This may involve short, frequent bouts of exercise and incorporating rest periods as needed.

6. Emphasizing Mind-Body Practices:

- Integrating mind-body practices such as yoga, meditation, or tai chi can be valuable for managing stress, improving mental health, and fostering a sense of well-being. These practices provide not only physical benefits but also emotional support during a challenging time.

7. Monitoring and Adjusting the Plan:

- Regular monitoring of the patient's response to the fitness routine is crucial. Adjustments should be made based on their comfort level, energy levels, and any emerging health concerns. Open communication with healthcare providers ensures that the fitness plan aligns with the ongoing medical treatment and recovery process.

8. Encouraging Social Support:

- Exercise can be more enjoyable and sustainable when shared with others. Encouraging cancer patients to engage in fitness activities with friends, family, or support groups fosters a sense of community and provides emotional support throughout their journey.

9. Staying Hydrated and Well-Nourished:

- Proper hydration and nutrition play pivotal roles in supporting overall health, particularly for individuals undergoing cancer treatment. Integrating guidance from a registered dietitian ensures that the fitness plan aligns with nutritional needs and supports recovery.

10. Fostering a Positive and Realistic Mindset:

- A positive mindset is crucial for navigating the challenges of cancer and fitness routines. Setting realistic goals, celebrating small achievements, and acknowledging the connection between physical and mental well-being contribute to a holistic and empowering approach.

CONCLUSION

In conclusion, "The Cancer-Fighting Diet" book not only serves as a valuable guide but also stands as a testament to the importance of holistic approaches in cancer prevention and overall well-being. The carefully curated content covers a diverse array of topics, ranging from nutrient-rich foods, antioxidants, and phytochemicals to the role of exercise in cancer prevention and tailored fitness routines for cancer patients.

The dietary recommendations provided emphasize the power of natural, whole foods, such as fruits, vegetables, whole grains, lean proteins, and fatty fish. These nutrient-dense choices are not only delicious but are backed by scientific evidence showcasing their potential in reducing the risk of cancer and promoting optimal health. By highlighting the unique properties of various food groups, the book empowers readers to make informed and positive choices in their dietary habits.

Furthermore, the inclusion of exercise as a fundamental component of cancer prevention is both insightful and actionable. The discussion delves into how regular physical activity can influence hormone levels, enhance immune function, and contribute to overall well-being. The tailored fitness routines for cancer patients provide a compassionate and individualized approach, recognizing the diverse challenges these individuals face and offering practical strategies for incorporating exercise into their lives.

The book's comprehensive exploration of cancer-fighting strategies goes beyond dietary recommendations and fitness routines. It underscores the importance of a positive mindset, community support, and the integration of mind-body practices in the journey to prevent and cope with cancer. By acknowledging the unique needs of each individual and promoting a human-centric approach, the book stands as a beacon of empowerment, guiding readers toward healthier and more resilient lives.

In essence, "The Cancer-Fighting Diet" is not just a collection of information but a holistic roadmap for individuals seeking to take charge of their health. It bridges the gap between scientific insights and practical, actionable steps, making the journey toward cancer prevention and recovery accessible, empowering, and ultimately transformative. Through these pages, readers are encouraged not only to embrace healthier dietary habits and exercise routines but also to cultivate a positive and resilient mindset that serves as a foundation for a life filled with vitality and well-being.

ABOUT THE BOOK

"Dive into 'The Cancer-Fighting Diet,' a transformative guide blending science-backed nutrition insights, empowering fitness strategies, and compassionate support for cancer patients. From nutrient-rich foods to tailored fitness routines, this book is your key to a resilient, health-focused journey. Elevate your well-being and embrace a holistic approach to cancer prevention with practical, human-centric wisdom."